YOUR KNOWLEDGE HAS VALUE

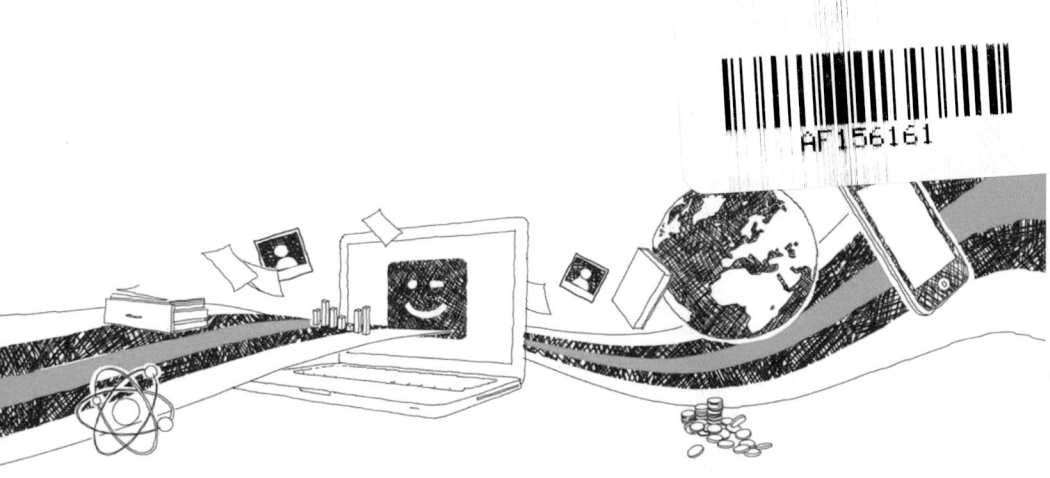
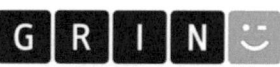

Bibliographic information published by the German National Library:

The German National Library lists this publication in the National Bibliography; detailed bibliographic data are available on the Internet at http://dnb.dnb.de .

Imprint:

Copyright © 2017 GRIN Verlag
Print and binding: Books on Demand GmbH, Norderstedt Germany
ISBN: 9783346022004

This book at GRIN:

https://www.grin.com/document/500560

Nadiia Kudriashova

Healthcare-associated Infections. Policy Analysis

GRIN Verlag

GRIN - Your knowledge has value

Since its foundation in 1998, GRIN has specialized in publishing academic texts by students, college teachers and other academics as e-book and printed book. The website www.grin.com is an ideal platform for presenting term papers, final papers, scientific essays, dissertations and specialist books.

Visit us on the internet:

http://www.grin.com/

http://www.facebook.com/grincom

http://www.twitter.com/grin_com

Healthcare-associated Infections: Policy Analysis

Healthcare-associated Infections: Policy Analysis

Nosocomial infections, having arisen at the dawn of the first medical institutions, became an increasingly complex and urgent problem of medicine. In modern conditions, the incidence of nosocomial infections, to a certain extent, reflects the quality of medical care provided to the population and is one of the important components of economic damage in practical health care.

According to research conducted by a single methodology under the auspices of WHO in fourteen countries, an average 8% of hospitalized patients infections are infected with with nosocomial infections. In the European region, the incidence of nosocomial infections is more than 7%, in the United States - about 5%; mortality is 2.7% (El-Saed, Balkhy, & Weber, 2013). The most common variants of nosocomial infections include nosocomial pneumonia, urinary tract infections, catheter-associated infections, and pseudomembranous colitis, or antibiotic-associated diarrhea. It should be understood that the localization of nosocomial infection depends on both the etiology of the pathogen and the source of nosocomial infections. Approximately 1 in 10 cases ends in death (Boev & Kiss, 2016). However, at least half of the infections are preventable. Policies and programs to combat nosocomial infections are aimed at this prevention.

In the structure of hospital mortality, nosocomial infections occupy the fourth place after diseases of the cardiovascular system, malignant tumors, acute disorders of cerebral circulation. The mortality of patients with nosocomial infection is almost two to three times higher in comparison with similar groups without this complication (Tawfiq & Tambyah, 2014). However, nowadays, few medical workers will dare to talk about the problem of nosocomial infection out loud and name the actual number of healthcare-associated infections in their medical institution, for fear of sanctions from regulatory bodies (Stone et al., 2015).

The lack of a unified approach to the identification of patients with nosomial infections in medical institutions, poor-quality organization of micro-biological monitoring, concealment of cases of healthcare-associated infections led to the fact that the registered incidence rate does not correspond to the actual one, which does not allow the hospital epidemiologist to carry out high-quality epidemiological diagnostics and targeted prevention. Meanwhile, nosocomial infections, in modern conditions, should be considered as a problem of the quality of treatment, the safety of medical care in a medical institution, and an important socio-economic problem.

Despite the fairly extensive information on nosocomial infections, it is difficult to get a true idea of the level, structure, and dynamics of the development of nosocomial infections and their epidemiological features. However, available information suggests that there is no tendency to reduce infections associated with the provision of medical care (Gomes et al., 2016). The need to improve the quality of medical care requires the development of a scientifically based set of preventive and anti-epidemic measures.

At the present stage, there are certain difficulties in combating nosocomial infections due to the presence of a large number of sources of infectious agents, their ways of transmission, high pathogen resistance to the effects of adverse environmental factors, variability of clinical manifestations, difficulty diagnosing individual nosological forms of nosocomial infection, and as a result - the lack of effective methods of specific prevention. All this does not allow effective impact on any link in the epidemic process.

The epidemiological surveillance program in each specific health facility must be adapted to the specific features of the institution. According to American researchers, an effective epidemiological surveillance program, given the current level of knowledge and technology, can prevent about one-third of all cases of nosocomial infection. However, if it is possible to achieve at least a 6% reduction in the level of nosocomial infections, the costs of this program pay off. The high incidence of nosocomial infections should not be considered as an excuse to punish the medical staff of a medical institution. In this case, it is necessary to look for the cause in the system of organization of epidemiological surveillance and make the necessary adjustments to it (El-Saed, Balkhy & Weber, 2013).

A new study has demonstrated how the risk of catching a nosocomial infection is changing with each day spent in an inpatient hospital at an American hospital. Researchers at South Carolina Medical University (MUSC) analyzed historical data from their academic medical center. The analysis included 949 cases of infection of patients with Gram-negative bacterial flora in the hospital, registered for the entire time of work. Scientists have discovered that the patient's chances of becoming infected with a multi-resistant gram-negative bacterial infection during treatment increase by an average of 1% for each day in the hospital. In their study, MUSC staff estimated that, in the first few days of hospitalization, about 20% of infections are associated with multi-resistant gram-negative bacteria. This percentage grows steadily in the first 4-5 days, and by the 10th day, it reaches 35%. After conducting a statistical analysis, the team concluded that the risk of multi-resistant gram-negative infections increases by 1% for each day of hospital stay. Professor John Bosso, from MUSC, says the data indicate the danger of nosocomial persistent infections. Statistics show that, at a minimum, unnecessary hospitalizations and unreasonably long hospitalizations should be avoided (Amin & Deruelle, 2015).

According to the US Centers for Disease Control and Prevention, gram-negative bacteria represent a very serious problem for American health care. They often cause severe postoperative infections, pneumonia, sepsis, meningitis. It is becoming increasingly obvious and frightening their growing resistance to widely used and most affordable antibiotics. Gram-negative bacteria acquire resistance to antibiotics through several mechanisms. They can transmit mutations to new generations, so resistance is quickly fixed and a new strain of bacteria appears that cannot be treated. The authors of the study say that nosocomial infections are responsible for a significant percentage of hospitalized patient deaths, and this percentage is increasing year by year (instead of decreasing due to the introduction of new antibiotics and antiseptic methods) (Shang et al., 2015).

Every day in the United States, 1 in 25 inpatients in US hospitals becomes infected a nosocomial infection, more than 30% of which are caused by Gram-negative bacteria. However, today, there is not enough information about how many infections and deaths are caused by this flora. The CDC estimates that in 2016, out of 722,000 ill patients, 75,000 people died from nosocomial infections. Over 50% of these deaths are recorded outside the intensive care unit (Zimlichman et al., 2013).

In the United States, the Active Bacterial Core Surveillance / Emerging Infections Program Network was developed in collaboration between the CDC, several state health departments, and universities. This program examines incidence trends in several states using molecular and microbiological antibiotic resistance testing methods for Streptococcus pneumoniae, Streptococcus pyogenes, Streptococcus agalactiae, Neisseria meningitidis, and Haemophilus influenzae (Boev & Kiss, 2016). Pharmaceutical companies, such as Alexander Project, MYSTIC, SENTRY, and TRUST are also often sponsors of antibiotic resistance research. The programs funded by the US government include the National Nosocomial infection surveillance system (NNIS), which conducts a study on antibiotic resistance in intensive care units in part of the hospitals participating in this system. However, up to 2 million cases of nosocomial infection are registered annually in US hospitals, in the structure of which 35% are accounted for purulent-septic infections (Amin & Deruelle, 2015).

To date, there are no standardized forms of accounting and a developed nomenclature of nosocomial infections that meets the requirements of WHO, which causes regular difficulties in registering and accounting for this group of diseases. The United States Centers for Disease Control and Prevention (CDC) distinguishes several major modes of transmission, depending on the isolation and restrictive measures that are required to protect patients and health care workers in particular transmission routes. Thus, the CDC classification is based on purely practical considerations and ignores some biologically significant transmission mechanisms that are rarely faced in the hospital and do not require special isolation-restrictive measures (Ellingson et al., 2014). For a long time, the concept of "nosocomial infections" was attributed only to infections and diseases in hospitals. Namely, this part of the nosocomial infection, the most significant in scale, attracted the attention of the health services in the first place. Of fundamental importance was the inclusion in the number of nosocomial infections in the 70s of all diseases associated with infection in hospitals, regardless of where the signs of the disease appeared and where nosocomial infection was diagnosed - in the hospital or after discharge. Currently, diseases of patients associated with the provision of medical care not only in hospitals, but also in any medical and preventive treatment institutions (polyclinic, medical unit, health center, ambulance) are classified as nosocomial infections. The breadth of distribution of these nosocomial infections is not well understood. The number of nosocomial infections, in addition to the diseases of patients, also includes diseases of medical workers. This aspect of the problem is the least studied (El-Saed, Balkhy, & Weber, 2013).

The lack of a full account and registration of nosocomial infection does not allow revealing the main causes of infection foci in a timely manner, makes it difficult to carry out in-depth analysis of the incidence, necessary to ascertain the conditions and nature of the epidemic process. Unfortunately, today, there is no single unified document containing important information for epidemiological analysis.

There are infection control departments in US hospitals. The staff is made of epidemiologists and nurses who have been trained in infection control at special courses. The nurses are taken to the department if they have at least ten years of experience; then they are assigned to the most experienced nurse of the infection control department, and only after completing the internship, the employee of the department has the right to work independently. The work is based on the principle of supervision of the departments (1 employee for 250 beds), collecting information, and analyzing cases of nosocomial infections. The data obtained as a result of this analysis is communicated to the department staff and discussed with it. However, there have been no significant improvements in the prevention of nosocomial infections (Stone et al., 2015).

The materials obtained in recent years indicate that nosocomial infections significantly prolong the length of stay of patients in hospitals and that the damage they cause annually in the United States ranges from 5 to 10 billion dollars (Zimlichman, 2013).

Describing the nosocomial infection, it should be noted that this category of infections has its specific characteristics of epidemiology, distinguishing it from the so-called "classic" infections. They are expressed in the peculiarities of the mechanisms and factors of transmission, the characteristics of the epidemiological and infectious processes, as well as in the fact that in the occurrence, maintenance, and spread of nosocomial infection foci, the medical personnel of the health care facilities - a relatively small part of the population - plays very significant role.

In matters of prevention of nosocomial infections in hospitals, junior and middle staff (nurses) are given the main leading role - the role of the organizer, the responsible executor, as well as the control function. Daily, thorough, and rigorous fulfillment of the requirements of the sanitary-hygienic and anti-epidemic regime in the course of fulfilling their professional duties forms the basis of the list of measures for the prevention of nosocomial infection (Gomes et al., 2016).

Speaking about the importance of the prevention of nosocomial infection, it should be noted that this problem is, certainly, complex and multifaceted. Each of the directions for the prevention of nosocomial infections involves some targeted sanitary and hygienic and anti-epidemic measures aimed at preventing a particular route of transmission of the infectious agent inside the hospital and should be considered separately. Such areas include general requirements for sanitary maintenance of premises, equipment, personal hygiene of patients and medical personnel, organization of disinfection practice, anti-epidemic requirements for presterilization processing and sterilization of medical products.

Disinfection is a very important area of prevention of nosocomial infection. This aspect of the activity of medical personnel is multicomponent and has as its goal the destruction of pathogenic and conditionally pathogenic microorganisms in the external environment of the wards and the functional premises of the hospital departments, medical instruments, and equipment. The organization of the disinfection practice and its implementation by the nursing staff is a complex, time-consuming daily duty.

Currently, there is a need to develop and implement control over the resistance of microorganisms that are the causative agents of nosocomial infection to disinfectants and antiseptics, in the framework of microbiological monitoring. To effectively conduct epidemiological surveillance in hospitals, it is preferable to have special hospital bacteriological laboratory, since this helps to ensure operational tripartite communication: a clinician - an epidemiologist - a bacteriologist. The funds spent on the laboratory will be reimbursed by the rational use of antibiotics, prevention of the formation of resistant hospital strains, effective control of nosocomial infections. The measures to improve the sanitary-hygienic and anti-epidemic regimes in the prevention of nosocomial infections in hospitals of various profiles also have not lost their significance.

The problem of prevention of nosocomial infection is multifaceted and is very difficult to be solved by some reasons - organizational, epidemiological, scientific, and methodological. The effectiveness of the fight against nosocomial infection is determined by the construction of health facilities according to the latest scientific achievements, their modern equipment and strict compliance with the requirements of the anti-epidemic regime at all stages of patient care. In hospitals, regardless of the profile, three essential requirements must be met: to minimize the possibility of infection being carried; eliminate intrahospital infections; exclude infection from the hospital.

Epidemiological surveillance should be carried out in each medical organization, taking into account its profile. Epidemiological surveillance in any medical organizations is organized and monitored by a hospital epidemiologist. The practice of the hospital epidemiologist shows that the epidemiological supervision and control of the nosocomial infection is characterized by high efficiency indicators in those medical organizations where the staffing position of the deputy chief physician on epidemiological issues is included in the staff list (Rahimi et al., 2017).

Evaluation of the activities carried out can be fulfilled using KPI indicators. Proper formation of the KPI system allows determining in which process the problem arose. The system of calculating KPI in health care meets the optimal criteria for a comprehensive assessment of activities: it has few indicators, which allows calculating KPIs on a monthly basis; the indicators have a quantitative characteristic and are objective. The definition of KPI should be based on their characteristics. The following characteristics of effective KPI are distinguished: Targeted belonging; Clear focus on results; Reachability; Openness to action; Providing forecasting activities; Limitations; Ease of perception by performers; Balance and interconnectedness; Initiation of change; Easiness to measure; Reinforcement with appropriate individual incentives; Relevance; Compatibility (Rahimi et al., 2017).

As a result of the implementation of the above measures, the overall economic effect achieved as a result of the implementation of the program - improving the efficiency of the business processes of the medical institution - should lead to an increase in revenue from the provision of services and increase profits. Identification of processes, employees, services that are not profitable for an institution contributes to cost reduction, growth of clinic profitability. There is an increase in control and improvement in the manageability of the hospital work as a whole, while maintaining or even reducing labor costs. As a result, the competitiveness of the clinic increases.

At the same time, non-observance of the proposed principles will obviously lead to the consolidation and worsening of the negative situation with the scale of nosomial infections dissemination and their consequences, and, accordingly, a gradual but tangible reduction in patient loyalty, complication of relations with insurance companies and contractors, as well as reduced attractiveness for potential investors.

At the same time, a conscientious attitude and the careful fulfillment by the medical staff of the requirements of the anti-epidemic regime will prevent the occupational morbidity of employees, which will greatly reduce the risk of infection and preserve the health of the patients.

References

Amin, A.N. & Deruelle, D. (2015). Healthcare-associated infections, infection control and the potential of new antibiotics in development in the USA. *Future Microbiology*, 10(6), 1049-1062.

Boev, C. & Kiss, E. (2016). Hospital-Acquired Infections. *Critical Care Nursing Clinics of North America,* 29(1), 51-65.

Casey, M. et al. (2015). Evidence-Based Programs and Strategies for Reducing Healthcare-Associated Infections in Critical Access Hospitals. *Flex Monitoring Team*, Policy Brief No. 40.

El-Saed, A., Balkhy, H.H., & Weber, D.J. (2013). Benchmarking local healthcare-associated infections: available benchmarks and interpretation challenges. *Journal of Infection and Public Health*, 6(5), 323-330.

Ellingson, K. et al. (2014). Enhancement of health department capacity for health care-associated infection prevention through Recovery Act-funded programs. *American Journal of Public Health*, 104, e27–e33.

Emerson, C.B. et al. (2012). Healthcare-associated infection and hospital readmission. *Infection Control & Hospital Epidemiology*, 33 (6), 539-544.

Gomes, A. et al. (2016). Prevention and Control of Infection: An Advanced Nursing Practice. *International Journal of Nursing*, 3(1), 81-88.

Rahimi, H. et al. (2017). Key performance indicators in hospital based on balanced scorecard model. *Journal of Health management & Informatics*, 4(1), 17-24.

Shang, J. et al. (2015). Studies on Nurse staffing and Healthcare Associated Infection: Methodological Challenges and Potential Solutions. *American Journal of Infection Control*, 43(6), 581-588.

Spruce, L. (2014). Featured article: back to basics: preventing surgical site infections. *The Association of periOperative Registered Nurses (AORN) Journal*, 99, 600–611.

Stone, P.W. et al. (2015). Impact of laws aimed at healthcare-associated infection reduction: a qualitative study. *BMJ Quality & Safety*, 24(10), 637-644.

Tawfiq, J. & Tambyah, P. (2014). Healthcare associated infections (HAI) perspectives. *Journal of Infection and Public Health*, 7(4), 339-244.

Zimlichman, E. et al. (2013). Health Care-Associated Infections: A Meta-analysis of Costs and Financial Impact on the US Health Care System. *JAMA*, 173(22), 2039-2046.

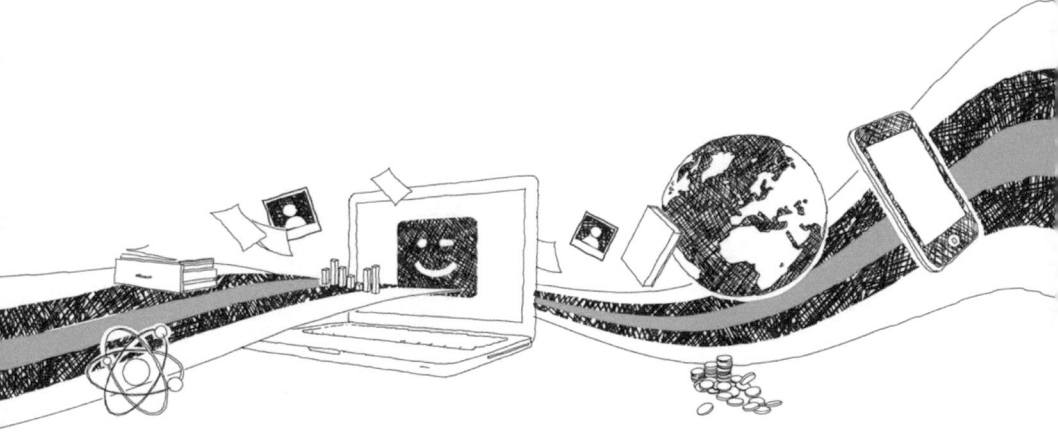
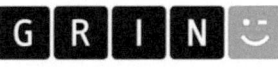